# The Wonder of DASH Diet

The No-Fluff Guide to Lowering High Blood Pressure, Losing Weight Fast, & Improving Health with the DASH Diet - Delicious Recipes & Meal Plan Included

Annabel W. Williams
Copyright© 2015 by Annabel W. Williams

# The Wonder of DASH Diet

Publisher: Living Plus Healthy Publishing

ISBN-13: 978-1517465582

ISBN-10: 1517465583

# Disclaimer

The Publisher has strived to be as accurate and complete as possible in the creation of this book. While all attempts have been made to verify information provided in this publication, the Publisher assumes no responsibility for errors, omissions, or contrary interpretation of the subject matter herein. Any perceived slights of specific persons, peoples, or organizations are unintentional.

This book is not intended for use as a source of legal, business, accounting or financial advice. All readers are advised to seek services of competent professionals in the legal, business, accounting, and finance fields.

The information in this book is not intended or implied to be a substitute for professional medical advice, diagnosis or treatment. All content contained in this book is for general information purposes only. Always consult your healthcare provider before carrying on any health program.

# Table of Contents

# Introduction

The DASH diet, far from being a fad diet, was actually developed by the US National Institutes of Health as a way for some patients to have a lowered blood pressure without having to take medications.

The word DASH comes from "Dietary Approaches to Stop Hypertension" but it does so much more. It has been studied extensively and found that not only does the DASH diet lower blood pressure but it lowers the risk of heart disease, stroke, certain cancers, heart failure, diabetes and kidney stones. Weight loss is practically inevitable if you follow this diet, which is another boost. Not only do you get healthier but you get thinner as well.

The DASH diet is based on solid research. Patients who followed the diet in research studies did more than lower their salt intake as a way to lower blood pressure. They followed an eating plan rich in fruits, vegetables, low fat dairy, whole grains and lean meats, among other things. The combination of things is what lowered their blood pressure.

The DASH diet, because it has been so well researched and found to be so successful, has been recommended by many different US agencies and associations, including:

- The American Heart Association

- The US Guidelines for the treatment of High Blood Pressure

- The National, Heart, Lung and Blood Institute

- The Dietary Guidelines for Americans

- The USDA MyPyramid

In its simplest terms, the DASH diet recommends (for those on a 2000 calorie a day diet) that you eat 7-8 servings of whole grains, 4-5 servings of fruits, 4-5 servings of vegetables, 2-3 servings of low fat or nonfat dairy foods, less than two servings of lean meats, poultry or fish, 4-5 servings a week of nuts, legumes and seeds, and limited amounts of sweets or fatty foods. If you're a connoisseur of the Mediterranean diet, you'll note that it is contained within the confines of the DASH diet.

In short, the DASH diet can be considered an excellent model for eating healthy whether or not you have high blood pressure. You don't have to make separate food for yourself and different food for your family. Everyone can benefit from eating this type of diet, even if they don't have any weight to lose or any history of hypertension.

So how does the DASH diet work? It certainly provides you with more nutrients than the average American diet and it is rich in minerals such as calcium, potassium and magnesium—all of which are known to reduce a person's blood pressure. You also have the option of reducing sodium in your diet, which is known to increase blood pressure in those with hypertension.

The good news is that the DASH diet plan is very flexible and is meant to be part of what a person does to live a healthy lifestyle, which means to limit alcohol intake, increase the amount of physical exercise, quit smoking, lower blood pressure, lower cholesterol, and maintain a healthy weight.

The DASH diet is extremely easy to follow once you know the rules and which foods should be emphasized. You might want to know how to follow the DASH diet if you are diabetic, if you have very high blood pressure or if you have cancer. This guide will make it clear to you how you should proceed with this type of diet while having chronic diseases.

In this guide, you'll learn about high blood pressure and related diseases. You'll see why it is important to follow the elements of the DASH diet as part of what it takes to lower blood pressure and maintain good health.

By the time you finish this guide, you will be armed with all the information you'll need to eat better, live better and live longer.

# Chapter 1: Understanding Hypertension

Hypertension is also called "high blood pressure". It is a condition where the pressure inside your heart and blood vessels is too high. When the heart pumps, it exerts pressure against the arteries, much like the pressure of a fire hose. When the heart relaxes, there is still some pressure in the arteries but it is less because the heart isn't actively beating.

This is why there are always two numbers associated with blood pressure. There is a top number called the systolic blood pressure, which is the arterial pressure when the heart is having a beat. The bottom number is the diastolic blood pressure or the resting blood pressure within the arteries.

A normal blood pressure is less than 120/80 much of the time, meaning the systolic blood pressure is 120 mmHg and the diastolic blood pressure is 80 mmHg. Those with a blood pressure of 140/90 or greater have hypertension and those in between have what's known as "prehypertension". If you have certain diseases, such as diabetes or heart disease, your doctor would usually like to see your blood pressure numbers lower than that, at 120/70 or so.

High blood pressure is a dangerous thing to have. It is the leading reason behind people having cardiovascular disease throughout the world. Hypertension affects about 28-29 percent of the US population. In other countries, the prevalence of high blood pressure has been increasing so that about 972 million people throughout the world suffer from this condition.

While people are generally being treated for high blood pressure, there is evidence to suggest that the control rates are not optimal. In the US, for example, only about 1/3 of all hypertensive patients are adequately controlled by diet and medications. As you'll see later in this guide, you can achieve control with the DASH diet alone.

There are a number of causes of hypertension including having too much salt in your body, having kidney disease, having a disease of your blood vessels, having a disease of your nervous system and having elevated levels of certain body hormones, such as epinephrine.

High blood pressure tends to become more prevalent with age. This is because your arteries stiffen as you get older and your blood pressure rises. High blood pressure makes you have a greater chance of having the following diseases:

- Heart attack

- Stroke

- Kidney disease

- Heart failure

- Premature death

Risk factors for high blood pressure include the following:

- Being overweight or obese

- Being African American

- Being stressed and anxious much of the time

- Drinking more than one drink per day (women) and more than two drinks per day (men)

- Consuming too much salt in the diet

- Having diabetes

- Having a smoking history

- Having a family history of high blood pressure

While there are many different causes of hypertension, you can easily have hypertension with no known risk factors. In this situation, it is often called essential hypertension.

It is also possible to have high blood pressure because of another medical condition. These conditions cause what's known as "secondary hypertension". Secondary hypertension can be permanent or can go away when the initial medical condition goes away. These primary medical conditions that lead to high blood pressure include:

- Cushing's syndrome—a disease of the adrenal gland where it releases too much cortisol

- Pheochromocytoma—an adrenal gland disease in which it releases too much epinephrine

- Chronic kidney disease, which releases hormones that participate in high blood pressure

- Pregnancy-induced hypertension—also called preeclampsia or toxemia

- Certain medications: cold medication, migraine medication, diet pills, birth control pills

- Renal artery stenosis—a narrowing of the arteries that supply the kidneys

- Hyperparathyroidism—an elevation of the parathyroid hormone

**What are the symptoms of hypertension?**

Sadly, many people have no symptoms of high blood pressure and only discover their problem when they get their blood pressure checked at the pharmacy or the doctor's office. What this means is that the first sign you might have high blood pressure might be one of the complications of the disease, such as stroke or a heart attack.

Some signs you might have a dangerous form of hypertension called malignant hypertension include having a severe headache, nausea, vomiting, visual changes and nose bleeds.

### What are the tests for blood pressure?

The doctor will check your blood pressure using a sphygmomanometer. This is a device that includes a cuff that goes around your arm, a bulb that increases the pressure in the cuff of the device and a measuring device that shows what the pressure is as the sphygmomanometer is being inflated or deflated.

The person checking the blood pressure inflates the cuff until the pressure is above the expected blood pressure and then decreases the pressure slowly. As the device reaches the systolic blood pressure a beat is heard and this persists until the diastolic pressure is reached. When the beat starts is the systolic blood pressure and when it stops is the diastolic blood pressure. The difference between the two numbers is called the "pulse pressure".

The "beat" represents an actual coming together of the arterial wall when the blood travels through it during systole but collapses, giving a "beat" during diastole. When the cuff pressure is below the systolic blood pressure, there is no beat because the artery isn't collapsing during diastole. When the cuff pressure is higher than the systolic blood pressure, there is no beat because the artery is fully collapsed during systole and diastole.

Your doctor may have to check your blood pressure several times in order to make the diagnosis of high blood pressure. Blood pressure can fluctuate so checking the blood pressure at different times of the day and different days is a good idea. Some people get "white coat syndrome" so their blood pressure is high at the doctor's office but not at home. Checking the blood pressure at home is also a good idea. Practice checking your blood pressure at your doctor's office with a home-based cuff to make sure you can easily check it without error.

Because high blood pressure is more dangerous when associated with other unhealthy conditions, the doctor may also order an echocardiogram or ultrasound of the heart, an electrocardiogram or electrical measurement of the heart, a stress exercise test, tests of kidney disease and a cholesterol panel. The doctor will also do a complete physical exam, looking for the effects of blood pressure on the body such as eye changes or a rhythm change in the heart.

## What is the treatment of hypertension?

The idea behind treatment of high blood pressure is to get the systolic and diastolic pressures down to the normal range so as to avoid the secondary complications of the disease. Even if you have prehypertension, your doctor may make some suggestions as to what you can do to prevent yourself from getting full blown hypertension.

Non-pill treatments include:

- The DASH diet plan

- The taking in of extra potassium and extra water, which help reduce blood pressure

- Exercise which includes at least 30 minutes of moderate aerobic exercise per day

- Quit smoking by whatever means you can

- Decrease your sodium (salt) intake

- Drink less than one alcoholic drink (women) or less than two alcoholic drinks per day (men)

- Reduce stress in your life, through changing your lifestyle, practicing yoga or practicing meditation

- Get to a healthy body weight using whatever program works for you. Try to get to a body mass index of 25 or less. Your body mass index is your weight in pounds times 703 divided by your height in inches squared.

Get as much help from your healthcare provider as to what you need to do in order to achieve a normal blood pressure. If you have prehypertension, your doctor will likely not treat the condition with medications unless you have an underlying disease like diabetes or heart disease.

If you have hypertension, the doctors will use any number of medication choices. Some medications for high blood pressure include:

- Diuretics, which help the kidney remove salt and water from your bodies so that the blood pressure in the arteries is less.

- Beta blockers, which slow down the heart and decrease the force of the heart.

- ACE inhibitors, which relax the blood vessels so the pressure is less in the arteries.

- Angiotensin II receptor blockers (ARBs), which work similarly to ACE inhibitors.

- Calcium channel blockers, which lower blood pressure by stopping calcium from getting into the cells.

- Alpha blockers, which relax the blood vessels, keeping the pressure low.

- Centrally acting drugs, which act on the brain to reduce the blood pressure.

- Vasodilators, which significantly relax the blood vessels.

- Renin inhibitors, which relax the blood vessels by acting on the kidneys.

## What are side effects of blood pressure medications?

It all depends on the medication you are taking and some high blood pressure medications have more side effects than others. Common side effects include changes in bowel habits, light-headedness, cough, erectile dysfunction, nervousness, fatigue or lack of energy, headache, nausea, rash or change in weight.

Sometimes one medication is all it takes. Other times, you need to be on more than one medication to keep your blood pressure under control.

## What are the complications of high blood pressure?

High blood pressure can be a dangerous thing to have if left untreated. High blood pressure puts extra pressure on the large and delicate small blood vessels of the body, causing rupture of blood vessels and bleeding complications. It can aggravate atherosclerosis so that some areas of the body can get poor blood supply. The major complications you'll find with hypertension include:

- Aortic rupture, which is bleeding from the blood vessel that leads from the heart to the pelvis. An aortic arterial rupture has a high mortality rate, even with corrective surgery.

- Heart attack. When the high blood pressure is associated with high cholesterol, the blood vessels that supply the heart get cut off and the end result is a heart attack.

- Heart failure. When the heart continually has to pump against high pressure, the muscle itself can begin to fail so that blood backs up into the lungs.

- Chronic kidney disease. The kidneys have delicate arteries that filter the blood and that get damaged when the blood pressure is too high for too long.

- Peripheral vascular disease. This is when the arteries supplying the legs become narrowed by cholesterol plaques and arterial spasm, leading to a reduced blood supply to the legs. It becomes painful to walk and there is a risk of a necessary amputation to prevent gangrene in the legs.

- Stroke. This is perhaps one of the more common complications of hypertension. It can happen in one of three ways. You can get a bleeding artery from high blood pressure resulting in a "hemorrhagic stroke". You can also get narrowing of one of the large arteries leading to the brain resulting in an "ischemic stroke". You can get multiple small blockages deep within the brain called "lacunar infarcts".

- High blood pressure can damage the small, delicate arteries of the eye so that you have hemorrhages or blockages, resulting in visual defects.

In the next chapter, we'll talk about how diet, good or bad, affects your blood pressure. Blood pressure is very sensitive to what you

eat so it pays to know the relationships between diet and blood pressure.

# Chapter 2: The Effects of Diet on Hypertension

There are many different foods that have an effect on blood pressure. Some last for a short time, such as the stimulant effects of caffeine in tea and coffee. Others, such as salt, affect the blood pressure over the long haul. Because food and food contents have such a strong effect on the blood pressure, it's a good idea to know which foods you should stay away from and which foods are good for you if you have high blood pressure.

A diet should ideally be as balanced as possible. If you have high blood pressure, you should make sure that you pay attention to foods you should limit as well as foods to add extra of in your diet. Let's look at some foods:

- **Salt**. Blood pressure and salt are greatly related and there is evidence to suggest that people who have high blood pressure are more sensitive to salt than people without the disease. Too much salt in the wrong person and there can be an increased risk of heart attack and stroke There is some disagreement as to how much salt you should eat in your diet; suffice it to say that if something tastes salty to you, it probably contains too much salt. Avoid things like potato chips, popcorn, canned soups and bacon, among other things. Don't add salt to your food.

- **Caffeine**. Caffeine is a stimulant food and medication. It increases the heart rate, blood pressure, metabolic rate and excites the nervous system. While the effects are usually only temporary, there are certainly long term effects of caffeine intake that may interest you. High caffeine consumption on a regular basis has been linked to high blood pressure in certain sensitive people. Other people seem to be extra-sensitive to caffeine and can get high blood pressure from even small amounts of caffeine. There are some people relatively resistant to the stimulatory effects of caffeine but there's no way to determine what category of people you fall into.

- **Alcohol**. It turns out that drinking one drink of alcohol per day for women and up to two alcoholic beverages per day for men can actually protect one from high blood pressure and its complications of heart attack, stroke and kidney disease. The alcohol makes the arterial walls more elastic so they respond differently to the various stress hormones when compared to people who do not drink alcohol. This results in an average low blood pressure and a decrease in the heart work load. Excessive alcohol, on the other hand, has the opposite effect on blood vessels. High alcohol content increases the stiffness of the arteries, increases the risk of metabolic "stress" in the system and makes the heart work harder.

- **Folic Acid**. Folic acid is the same thing as synthetic B9 and it is fortified in foods like flour, bread and cereals. There is good evidence to suggest that folic acid is good for lowering blood pressure and can block the onset of high blood pressure when taken in amounts that are approximately 800 micrograms per day. Interestingly, this excellent effect of folic acid on high blood pressure has only been observed in female subjects of research studies. The research on men is less well studied but it is recommended that men take in about 400 micrograms of folic acid per day. For those with high blood pressure, however, it may be a good idea to increase the daily content of folic acid to 800 micrograms per day, whether or not you are male or female.

- **Potassium**. Too little potassium in your diet and your blood pressure will go up, putting you at an increased for stroke. This finding has been noted in research studies with both humans and animals. Potassium is a chemical messenger that works with other ions and chemicals in the body to keep the blood vessels relaxed and supple. This lowers blood pressure when taken in at 40 mEq per day. One good way to get potassium in your diet is to purchase salt substitute, which salts items you're eating leading to a salty flavor but with the benefits of potassium instead.

- **Magnesium**. Magnesium in the diet has been known to have similar effects on blood pressure as does Potassium; however, the research is less clear. While it has already been shown that an excess of Magnesium definitely lowers blood pressure, no one knows yet if a lack of magnesium in the diet causes high blood pressure. These are studies that have yet to be performed. Even so, extra magnesium in your diet seems to be good for you and will help reduce your blood pressure.

- **Vitamin D**. Vitamin D is useful as part of managing the regulatory functions of the body. It contributes to the amount of Calcium in the bloodstream, which, in turn, reduces the blood pressure. Research has shown that having a vitamin D deficiency can cause high blood pressure. Vitamin D deficiency is common in those areas of the world that have long and dark winters with little individual sun exposure. Other heart problems have been associated with low vitamin D levels. Fortunately, many foods you eat are already fortified with vitamin D.

- **A healthy high blood pressure diet**. If you find yourself with high blood pressure, you will do yourself some good to eat a low fat diet with plenty of fruits and vegetables and low amounts of sweets and red meat.

- **Whole grains**. These are particularly good for lowering blood pressure. Some of the best sources of whole grains include natural oat products, barley and whole grain breads. As complex carbohydrates, whole grains are great long term sources of energy. They help manage high cholesterol and keep sudden fluctuations of insulin at bay. Whole grains help you reduce your appetite so you stand a better chance of maintaining a healthy weight. This also reduces blood pressure.

- **Fruits and Vegetables**. These are loaded with healthy vitamins and excellent sources of stable energy and fiber.

Fruits and vegetables are low in calories so, when they curb your appetite, they also help you maintain a healthy weight. Whole fruits are much preferable to fruit juices as the whole fruit will help regulate the blood pressure and lower blood cholesterol levels. Try to eat three different colored vegetables with each meal, such as orange carrots, tomatoes and green beans. You're better off if you steam vegetables or eat them raw as opposed to boiling them.

- **Lean Meats**. Meats aren't off the list in a healthy diet as long as they are meats with very little fat content in them. You can find lean meat sources in fish, lean pork and poultry. You can also explore the very lean meats of ostrich and buffalo meat. Buffalo, for example, has a taste just like beef but contains only half the fat and a third of the calories of white meat poultry. Overall, you should limit the number of servings of meat you eat per day but once in a while won't hurt you.

- **Fats**. Both saturated fats and trans fats are terrible for your blood vessels, your blood pressure and your heart. These are the fats that clog your arteries and make the blood have to sneak through ever narrower lumens. Saturated fats and trans fats should simply be off your diet if you have high blood pressure unless it's for a rare, special occasion. High blood pressure and fatty arteries are a recipe for disaster.

In the next chapter, we'll introduce the DASH diet, which incorporates a lot of these foods known to help lower blood pressure and you'll see how you can eat without dipping into the foods or food ingredients that make blood pressure worse.

# Chapter 3: The DASH Diet

By now, hopefully you're convinced that food and high blood pressure are related. This is what those that designed the DASH Eating Plan also determined. With that knowledge in mind, they created a diet plan for those who not only have high blood pressure but for those who are at high risk for high blood pressure. In fact, the combination of eating the DASH diet and lowering the dietary consumption of salt can have the best benefit when it comes to preventing or lowering blood pressure.

In this chapter, you'll learn how to start eating the DASH diet and how to remain on the diet plan for years to come. Later, we'll talk about recipes and meal plans. Each meal plan on the DASH diet has around 1500-2300 milligrams of sodium per day. The value of 2300 milligrams is the most sodium allowable by the National High Blood Pressure Education Program and the highest recommended amount as listed by the "US Dietary Guidelines for Americans" from 2005. Suffice it to say that the lower the sodium level in your diet, the better your blood pressure should be.

As for salt, the average sodium content in today's American diet is about 4200 milligrams per day for men and 3300 milligrams per day for women. It appears that everyone could stand to reduce sodium to a level that would improve blood pressure. That and the DASH diet should help many in America avoid having to take antihypertensive medications.

## Quick Facts of the DASH Diet Plan

The higher your blood pressure rises above 120/80, the greater is your risk of secondary hypertensive complications like stroke, heart attack, eye damage or kidney damage. This has clearly been supported by the experts at the National, Heart, Lung and Blood Institute or NHLBI. The experts also showed that eating the food recommended in the DASH plan not only lowered blood pressure but had positive effects on cholesterol numbers in the bloodstream.

The DASH eating plan can lower your blood pressure by eating certain amounts of fruits, vegetables, low fat or fat free dairy products, whole grain products and small amounts of nuts, fish and poultry. It is a diet rich in healthy magnesium, calcium and potassium—all of which lower blood pressure. This is a diet that eliminates red meat, added sugar, sugary beverages and sweets that are so commonly found in today's American diet.

The daily nutrient goals include the following:

- Potassium—at least 4700 mg

- Sodium—no more than 2300 mg

- Magnesium levels—no less than 500 mg

- Calcium—at least 1250 mg

- Total fat no greater than 27 percent of calories

- Saturated fat no greater than 6 percent of calories

- Carbohydrates at least 55 percent of calories

- Cholesterol 150 mg or less

- Fiber at least at 30 grams per day

For those who are at least middle aged, the recommendations for sodium go down to 1500 mg per day. The same is true for African Americans and for those who already suffer from hypertension.

The first study to evaluate the DASH diet looked at almost 500 adults who had blood pressures of less than 160 mmHg systolic and no more than 95 mg diastolic. About 1/4 of all these people already suffered from hypertension. The study compared a regular American diet, a regular American diet plus added fruits and vegetables and the DASH plan. All three diets had 3,000 mg of sodium in the diet.

The results showed that both those people who ate more fruits and vegetables and those on the DASH diet had lower blood pressure; however, those on the DASH diet did the best, particularly for those who already had hypertension. The results worked well within 2 weeks of beginning the diet.

The second DASH research study looked at what sodium has to do with the diet. About 400 participants followed the DASH diet or a typical American diet. There were those who ate 3300 mg of sodium per day; there were those that ate 2300 mg of sodium per day; some took in only 1500 mg of sodium per day. At each level of sodium intake, the DASH diet did better than the American diet. The higher blood pressures were reduced the most on a low sodium diet. Basically, the researchers concluded that the DASH diet plus sodium reduction are what's necessary when it comes to improving the blood pressure.

The DASH diet doesn't really count calories. Rather, it assumes a caloric content of about 2000 mg per day and gives you the number of servings of each type of food to be used each day. The DASH diet also gives you the number of servings to eat per day on a 1600, 2600 and 3200 calorie per day diet plan.

This is the food group servings you should eat per day on a 2000 calorie per day plan:

## Grains

- Serving Size: 1 slice bread, 1 oz cereal
- Number of Servings: 6-8

## Vegetables

- Serving Size: 1 cup raw leafy veg., 1/2 cup cut up veg.
- Number of Servings: 4-5

## Fruits

- Serving Size: 1 medium fruit, 1/4 cup dried fruit
- Number of Servings: 4-5

## Low fat dairy

- Serving Size: 1 cup milk or yogurt, 1.5 ounces cheese
- Number of Servings: 2-3

## Lean meats, poultry and fish

- Serving Size: 1 oz cooked meat, 1 egg
- Number of Servings: 6 or less

## Nuts, seeds and legumes

- Serving Size: 1/3 cup nuts, 1-1/2 oz nuts
- Number of Servings: 4-5 per week

## Fats and oils

- Serving Size: 1 tsp soft margarine, 1 tbsp mayonnaise
- Number of Servings: 2-3 per week

## Sweets and added sugar

- Serving Size: 1 tbsp jelly or jam, 1 cup lemonade
- Number of Servings: 5 or less per week

You need to pay close attention to portion size because portion sizes are generally much less than you actually eat. For example, if you eat a turkey sandwich with mayonnaise, you've already eaten two serving sizes of bread, at least one or more servings of turkey and a serving of fats and oils. And if you put more than just a tablespoon of mayonnaise on your sandwich, which is easy to do, you've eaten a whole week's worth of fats and oils.

## Which foods are allowed on this diet plan?

Technically, there is a large variety of things you can include on the DASH diet plan but these things can be used as a guide:

- **Grains**: Whole wheat bread, whole wheat rolls, English muffin, whole wheat pasta, oatmeal, brown rice, grits, bagels, cereals, popcorn, brown rice, and unsalted pretzels.

- **Vegetables**: Carrots, collard greens, broccoli, peas, green beans, lima beans, potatoes, spinach, sweet potatoes, kale, tomatoes, and squash.

- **Fruits**: Apricots, bananas, dates, apples, oranges, grapes, grapefruit juice and grapefruit, mangoes, raisins, melons, peaches, pineapples, tangerines and strawberries.

- **Nonfat/low fat dairy products**: Fat free milk, 1 percent milk, low fat buttermilk, low fat or fat-free cheese, low fat or fat-free yogurt.

- **Lean meat**: trimmed away poultry broiled, roasted or poached without skin and fish.

- **Nuts and legumes**: Hazelnuts, peanuts, almonds, mixed nuts, sunflower seeds, peanut butter, lentils, split peas and kidney beans.

- **Fats and oils**: Vegetable oil, soft margarine, low-fat mayonnaise, light salad dressing.

- **Sugar added**: Jell-O with sugar, hard candy, jelly, fruit punch, maple syrup, sorbet, ices, and sugar.

The DASH diet is a major source of healthy energy, fiber, magnesium, potassium, calcium and protein. The sweets you eat should be low in fat because they count as both sweet and fat servings. You should limit your egg yolk intake to no more than 4 per day. Two egg whites equal one ounce of meat.

You should try to achieve a normal weight with this diet. You can accomplish this by doing the DASH diet for 1600 calories instead of 2000. Even at 2000 calories per day, you can lose weight, albeit slowly.

One study looked at more than 800 people who participated in a study. One third of all patients were taught how to lower their salt intake and were instructed on the DASH diet. Many of these people needed to lose weight. After following the DASH diet and increasing their physical activity, most participants lost weight and improved their blood pressure after just 18 months.

You need to aim for eating fewer calories than you are currently eating and this is definitely something possible with the DASH diet. On a 1600 calorie a day diet, you'd eat the following number of servings:

- Grains—6 servings

- Vegetables—3-4 servings

- Fruits—4 servings

- Fat-free or low fat milk –2-3 servings

- Lean meats, Poultry, and fish—3-6 servings

- Nuts, seeds, and Legumes—3 servings per week

- Fats and oils—2 servings per week

- Sweets and added sugars—0 servings per week

Some low calorie, low fat tips include the following great weight loss recommendations:

- Eat a medium apple to increase fruits rather than eating cookies.

- Eat 1/4 cup dried apricots for a snack instead of a 2 ounce bag of pork rinds.

- Eat a 3 ounce hamburger instead of a 6 ounce hamburger.

- Add half cup carrots and half cup spinach instead of French fries or a baked potato.

- Instead of eating five oz of chicken, make a stir fry with just 2 oz of chicken and a cup and a half of raw vegetables with very little vegetable oil.

- To eat more low-fat dairy have a half cup of low fat frozen yogurt instead of the same amount of ice cream containing fat. You can save at least 70 calories.

- Use fat free condiments like mustard or ketchup instead of mayonnaise.

- Try to cook with half as much vegetable oil as you're used to. The same holds true for soft margarine and mayonnaise.

- Gradually decrease your portion size.

- Watch the fat content on food labels.

- Stay away from high sugar foods like flavored yogurt, cakes, pies, ice cream, sherbet, soft drinks, fruity drinks and candy bars.

- Add fruit to fat free plain yogurt as the sugar content is less.

- Eat fruit or vegetable sticks for snacks as well as unbuttered popcorn without salt.

- Drink more water or even club soda. Spice it up with a lime or lemon wedge.

If you are trying to lower your blood pressure and your weight at the same time, it might be a good idea to speak to your doctor and a dietician to get ideas on what to eat and how much exercise is safe for you. If your blood pressure is very high, you may still need to be on medication along with the DASH diet in order to keep both your weight and blood pressure low.

You should also notice that the DASH diet provides more fiber through grains, fruits and vegetables. More fiber can mean side effects of bloating and diarrhea in people not used to the change in dietary habits. If this happens to you, you should increase your intake of these fiber-causing foods slowly and gradually so that your intestines become used to the changes.

Remember that the DASH diet works much better if you also lower your salt intake. Actually, very few people really add a lot of salt to their diet through adding salt from a salt shaker. In addition, there is little salt in natural foods. This means that most salt gets in foods through cooking or processing.

If you eat processed food, read the food label so that you know how much food you're really getting in the product. At the same time you do this, you need to pay attention to the number of servings in the package. If you eat a can of soup that contains 2 servings and 900 milligrams of sodium per serving, if you eat the whole thing, you've eaten 1800 milligrams of sodium in one meal!

## Physical Activity

While the DASH diet is truly just a diet, there is ample evidence that this kind of diet works best when you eat it along with exercising on a regular basis. Exercise uses up calories so you can lose weight more effectively and it increases your metabolic rate so that you continue to burn calories at a greater rate even though you have stopped exercising.

Exercise can be walking, running, bicycling, swimming or other fun activity. You need to exercise for at least 10 minutes at a given time and for about 30 minutes per day. What's important is that you get the full thirty minutes of exercise in per day. If you're trying to lose weight actively, you should increase your activity level to about 60 minutes per day.

So how do you get into physical activity when you've been sedentary for a long period of time? One good way is to start walking for fifteen minutes twice a day—once before work in the morning and once in the evening. Build up your stamina by walking faster or longer each time. If you have an activity that is particularly enjoyable, like swimming or bicycling, do these activities instead. Don't push yourself too hard in the beginning or you will get injured and this might be too discouraging.

Your doctor should know about your physical activity if you have a personal or family history of heart disease. You might be a candidate for a stress exercise test of the heart to make sure it is safe for you to exercise.

What should you do?

- You should create an exercise schedule and stick with it.

- You should get a relative or friend to motivate you and join you in the activity.

- Try to cross-train. This involves switching up exercise types as you exercise.

- Set goals for yourself and try to reach them.

- Reward yourself for doing a good job on your exercise program.

## Keeping Salt out of Your Diet

It is, of course, important to keep salt out of your diet if you want to lower your blood pressure maximally. Here are some tips to lowering your salt intake:

- If there are low sodium versions of foods you like to eat, try to choose those versions rather than the higher salt varieties.

- Choose frozen or fresh vegetables as canned vegetables sometimes have too much salt.

- Use fresh lean meats, poultry or fish rather than smoked, processed or canned meats.

- Select those ready-to-eat breakfast cereals that are lowest in sodium per serving.

- Don't eat much bacon or ham as these are cured meats high in sodium.

- Eliminate foods packed in brine like olives, sauerkraut and pickled vegetables.

- Condiments like horseradish, mustard, barbecue sauce and ketchup are high in salt.

- Cook pasta, rice and hot cereals without salt. Cereal mixes and flavored pastas/rice usually have excess salt.

- Cut back on frozen dinners, packaged mixes and pizza, which are high in salt.

- Rinse out things like canned beans and tuna to get the sodium out of it.

- Make great use of spices that flavor your food without adding salt. There are a lot of herbs, spices and salt-free alternatives to flavoring your food.

## Potassium

One of the ideas behind the DASH eating plan is to increase the potassium content in the food. Potassium comes from fruits and vegetables and helps you to decrease your blood pressure. It's a good idea to get your potassium from food sources rather from a potassium supplement, although potassium supplements do exist and can be purchased from the grocery store. Some milk products and fish contain potassium as well.

What you're looking for is potassium with bicarbonate precursors that are good for your acid-base metabolism. This type of potassium also decreases the incidence of kidney stones and improves bone mass. Foods that contain potassium include:

Potatoes, Sweet Potatoes, Spinach, Zucchini, Tomato, Kale, Romaine Lettuce, Mushrooms, Cucumber, Banana, Apricots, Orange, Cantaloupe, Apple, Soybeans, Cooked lentils, Kidney beans, Split peas, Almonds, Walnuts, Sunflower seeds, Peanuts, Milk, Yogurt, Fish, Pork tenderloin, Beef tenderloin.

## Reading Labels

If you're going to be a savvy shopper of foods containing fats and sodium, you need to know what these labels mean. The following list gives you the meaning of various labels you will come across:

- **Salt-free or sodium-free**: Less than 5 mg sodium per serving.

- **Very low sodium**: 35 milligrams of sodium or less per serving.

- **Low sodium**: 140 mg of sodium or less per serving.

- **Low sodium meal**: 140 milligrams or less per 3-1/2 ounces

- **Reduced or less sodium**: At least 25 percent less sodium than the regular version

- **Light in sodium**: 50 percent less sodium than the regular version.

- **Unsalted or no salt added**: Product has had no extra salt added during processing.

- **Fat-free**: Less than a half gram per serving

- **Low saturated fat**: 1 gram or less per serving and 15 percent or less is saturated fat.

- **Low-fat**: Three grams or less per serving.

- **Reduced fat**: At least 25 percent less fat than the regular version.

- **Light in fat**: Half the fat of the regular version.

### So how do you get started with the DASH eating plan?

If you are thinking you might want to adopt the DASH Eating Plan but don't know how to start, make sure you start gradually. If you now eat a serving or two of vegetables per day, add two more servings. If you don't eat fruit, add a piece of fruit as an afternoon snack. Read labels and use fat free dairy products up to three times per day. Drink milk, for example, at dinner instead of sodas.

Always read nutrition labels and know how much sodium and fat you are taking in. When you eat meat, have the meat be only a small portion of the meal instead of the focus of the meal. This means using less meat on your plate. You really only need six ounces of meat each and every day. If you now eat a lot of meat, simply cut back gradually so you're not eating so much meat each day. Try some vegetarian meals. Try more vegetables, brown rice, cooked beans and cooked whole wheat pasta in your diet. Soon the DASH diet will be a normal thing for you and you'll know what to buy at the grocery store.

Write down what you're currently eating and do this for breakfast, lunch, dinner and snacks for one week. Keep track of the calories, servings, potassium, and sodium levels for that time. Find places where you can learn to make better choices.

## Tips for Eating Out

Eating out can be hard because restaurant food isn't designed to be healthy; it's designed to be especially rich and tasty. Here are some eating-out tips that will help you on the DASH diet.

- Know the terms, like cured, smoked, broth, soy sauce and pickled.

- Ask the waiter how food is prepared and ask if they can be prepared without MSG or added salt.

- Don't even think about the salt shaker.

- Really cut down on the different condiments, most of which contain too
  much salt.

- Choose fruits and vegetables as side
  dishes and limit any kind of salty snack
  foods like French fries.

- Portions tend to be large so cut everything in half, eat the half and take the
  rest home for another meal.

## Your DASH Goals

Your DASH goals, if you follow the plan
right will be accomplished. These goals are to
eat foods that lower your blood pressure, eat
foods low in sodium, eat foods high in potassium, drink alcohol in moderation, exercise at
least 30 minutes per day, and maintain a
healthy weight.

# Chapter 4: DASH Diet as Part of a Weight Loss Program

One of the goals of the DASH diet is to maintain a healthy weight. But what if you're not at a healthy weight and you would very much like to get there using the DASH diet. Actually, all the parameters are there for you to lose weight by following the number of servings of the different kinds of food for a 1600 calorie per day diet. You'll lose weight and you'll feel healthy as a result.

With the DASH diet, you'll be eating healthy foods based on fruits, vegetables and whole grains—all of which are low in fat and calories. You won't feel like you're starving yourself and you'll feel like you're eating very satisfying foods without overeating. According to recent research, the calcium you're getting in the diet aid the weight loss process.

Losing weight and reducing sodium in your diet will reduce your blood pressure and the complications that come with it like stroke, heart attack, kidney failure and peripheral vascular disease. In this chapter, we'll figure out exactly how much you should be weighing and we'll calculate the number of calories you'll need to lose the weight and reduce blood pressure.

Research on the DASH diet supports the idea that it can help with weight loss. Because the diet is rich in fruits and vegetables, it is filling without adding calories. It also makes use of lower fat meats, fish and poultry that have fewer calories than the high fat versions. Low fat dairy products are lower in calories and the calcium promotes weight loss.

It's well known that being overweight contributes to high blood pressure, especially in children and teens. If you adopt the DASH diet for the whole family, your children may also be spared obesity and high blood pressure complications. You can even exercise together.

## What should I weigh?

Years ago, in order to learn the weight you should be, you looked at the Metropolitan Life Weight Tables and they told you what to weigh. Now they have invented a thing called the BMI or Body Mass Index.

The Body Mass Index is based on your height and weight and is calculated as such: The BMI = weight in pounds x 703 divided by height in inches squared. Another indicator is the Body Fat Percentage. This is more difficult to calculate.

The normal body mass index is 19-25. If your BMI is less than 19, you are underweight. If the BMI is between 25 and 29.9, you are overweight. If the BMI is greater than 30, you are considered obese. If your weight yields a BMI of around 25 or less, this is a desirable weight. To calculate your healthy weight, use this formula: weight = 0.0456 x height squared.

While BMI is a good measurement, it doesn't tell you how much fat you have in your body so a muscled football player would look like he is overweight when he is completely physically fit. As mentioned, the Body Fat Percentage is a better measure of fat in your body but it's a difficult test to actually do.

The test for the body fat percentage can be done using a DEXA scan, which is the same test used for bone density. There is also an inexpensive BIA test or the bio-electric impedance analysis to test for body fat percentage. It is usually only done in research facilities. Weighing you underwater can tell you your body fat analysis and this is done sometimes at health clubs.

Waist size is another way to determine if you need to lose weight. This can tell you if you have most of your weight around your middle—a sure sign of increased risk of heart disease and stroke. Those people who are more pear-shaped have a lesser risk of heart disease. The waist circumference should be less than 35 inches in women and less than 40 inches in men. As you lose weight, you should see a reduction in your waist size.

### How much weight should I lose?

Research has shown that if you lose 7-10 percent of your body weight, you will experience a significant improvement in your blood pressure and health. If you feel like you have a long way to go before reaching a BMI of less than 25, you can set a short term goal to simply lose about 10 percent of your body weight.

When you lose weight, you should strive for 1-2 pounds per week in women and about

2-4 pounds per week for men. You'll lose more weight in the beginning and it gets harder when you've lost a portion of your weight. If you lose weight too fast, you will lose both muscle and fat and you don't want to be losing muscle as you diet.

In order to lose one pound per week, you need to reduce your caloric intake by 500 calories per day. One pound equals 3500 calories so after a week, you'll lose a pound. Look at your weekly diet plan and find ways to lose 500 calories per day.

You'll want to determine how many calories your body needs. It's completely related to your activity level and your weight. Use the following table to determine your calorie needs and remember that, as your weight decreases, your caloric allowance will decrease as well:

### Activity Level – Calories needed per Pound

- Sedentary – 13.5
- Moderate – 16
- Heavy – 18

Even when you lose weight, you should stay on the DASH diet because it will continue to lower your blood pressure and will keep you from suffering any of the complications of high blood pressure.

# Chapter 5: DASH Recipes

In this chapter, we will look at some great recipes that work well in the DASH diet and will finish with a 7 day sample meal plan. This will help you get a feel of the different kinds of foods you can eat with a DASH diet and know that the food will be helpful to your body.

## Breakfast Recipes

With the DASH diet, having a good breakfast in the morning is important to curb hunger throughout the morning and to get your metabolic rate jump started. Here are some good recipes to do this:

# Egg Muffins

## Ingredients:

- 1/4 cup diced onion
- 2 cup liquid egg substitute
- 1/4 cup finely chopped green pepper
- 16 oz. of frozen chopped spinach
- 3/4 cup low fat shredded mozzarella cheese

## Directions:

1. Place foil cups in a muffin pan. Spray the cups with cooking spray.

2. Microwave the frozen spinach for about 2.5 minutes. Allow to cool before squeezing out the liquid. Put the dried spinach in a mixing bowl.

3. Add green pepper, onion, egg, and cheese to bowl. Mix evenly.

4. Pour a fourth of a cup of mixture into each foil cup.

5. Bake at 350 degrees for 20 minutes or until a knife comes out clean.

6. 3 muffins equal one serving.

## Breakfast Pretzels

These are hearty and low in fat so they make a great breakfast choice.

### Ingredients:

- 1 tube of Pillsbury pizza crust dough
- 1/4 cup flour
- 1 beaten egg
- 2 tablespoons butter
- 1/4 cup brown sugar
- 1/4 cup powdered sugar

### Directions:

1. Spray a baking sheet with cooking spray.

2. Cut unrolled dough into 4 strips. Roll into a 16 inch rope. Make a pretzel out of it and place onto baking sheet.

3. Put all the dry ingredients together to make a streusel.

4. Brush the pretzels with the egg. Sprinkle the streusel on the pretzels.

5. Bake at 400 degrees for 20 minutes or until pretzels are golden brown.

6. One pretzel is one serving.

## Egg Tortillas

**Ingredients:**
- 4 flour tortillas
- 4 eggs
- 1/4 cup salsa
- 1/4 cup shredded cheese blend

**Directions:**

1. Use a microwave oven safe bowl and put a paper towel in it (lined).

2. Line the bowl with the tortilla and crack an egg in the middle.

3. Cook in the microwave for 30 seconds and then stir egg.

4. Cook for another 15-30 seconds.

5. Add cheese and salsa to the egg and wrap up the tortilla in the paper towel.

6. Repeat three more times for the rest of the tortillas.

7. One tortilla equals one serving.


## Breakfast Polenta with Brown Sugar

### Ingredients:

- 1 cup polenta (white or yellow corn-meal)
- 2 cup fat-free milk
- 1/2 tsp vanilla extract
- 1/2 tsp salt
- 1/4 cup brown sugar
- Pinch of cinnamon
- 3 cup cold water

### Directions:

1. Mix polenta with 1 cup of water in a small bowl. Stir and let sit.

2. In a medium saucepan, mix milk with 2 cup water. Slowly boil this mixture and add salt.

3. Slowly put in the polenta and water mixture. Whisk to mix well.

4. Reduce to low heat and simmer until polenta is thickened, between 10 and 40 minutes.

5. Add sugar, vanilla extract, and cinnamon.

6. Serves for 4.

## Lunch Recipes

Lunch ideally should be something you can make and eat at work, school or wherever you might be during the day. These are some healthy DASH lunch recipes:

## Lunch Lasagna

This is a good recipe to make the night before and then put in a large slice of the lasagna in a Tupperware container for lunch.

### Ingredients:
- 1 pound ground turkey, lean
- 1 large diced onion
- 1 cup grated carrots
- 1 large whisked egg
- 1 tbsp olive oil

- 2 jars of salsa
- 1 clove garlic, minced
- 1 tsp ground cumin
- 2 cup Mexican cheese, grated
- 1/2 tsp salt
- 1/2 tsp chili powder
- 1/2 cup lean sour cream
- 1/4 cup chopped cilantro
- 1 pkg corn tortillas (about 12)

**Directions:**

1. Sauté onions for three minutes in a small amount of olive oil. Add garlic and continue to sauté for another minute.

2. Add turkey, cumin, salt, and chili powder and cook the mixture until the chicken is cooked through, about 7 minutes. Let turkey mixture cool.

3. Mix egg and sour cream together and add carrots, corn, cilantro, and the turkey mixture.

4. Spread a cup of salsa in the bottom of a slow cooker.

5.  Layer five tortillas onto the salsa and then put half the turkey mixture on the tortillas.

6.  Add a cup of salsa and 1/2 cup cheese.

7.  Place three more tortillas on top of that and then put the rest of the turkey mixture on top of the tortillas.

8.  Add another 1/2 cup of cheese.

9.  Finish off with rest of tortillas, salsa and cheese.

10. Cook in slow cooker in low for 2.5 hours.

### Curried Potatoes

**Ingredients:**
- 1 pound small, new potatoes (about ten potatoes)
- 2 onions, finely chopped
- 1/2 cup chicken broth
- 1 clove garlic, minced
- 1 tsp curry powder
- 1/4 cup cilantro leaves, finely chopped
- 1/2 tsp salt
- 1/2 tsp black pepper

- 2 tbsp squeezed lemon juice

**Directions:**

1. Brown potatoes in a skillet sprayed with cooking spray or rubbed with a small amount of oil.

2. Transfer the potatoes to a slow cooker.

3. Place onions, garlic, salt, and pepper in skillet and sauté until softened.

4. Add broth and boil over the potatoes. Add onion mixture to potatoes.

5. Cook in slow cooker for 8 hours on low or for 4 hours on high.

6. Mix lemon juice & curry powder and add to potato mixture. Cook for 10 minutes on high heat.

7. Garnish with cilantro.

# Lunchtime Caesar Salad

**Ingredients:**

- 1 large egg
- 3 hearts of separated Romaine lettuce
- 3 tbsp grated Parmesan cheese
- 2 cloves of garlic, minced
- 1 tbsp Dijon mustard
- 1 tbsp of anchovies, minced
- 1/4 cup olive oil
- 2 tsp grated lemon zest
- 1 tbsp of red-wine vinegar
- 2 cup croutons
- Black pepper to taste

**Directions:**

1. Mix anchovies, garlic, lemon zest, mustard, and vinegar together.

2. Drizzle in olive oil & whisk until mixture is thick. Add pepper to taste and set aside.

3. Place lettuce in a large bowl. Toss it with about a third of the dressing mix.

4. Break the egg onto the salad. Serve with croutons and dressing on the side.

5. Serves 6.

## Chicken Salad

**Ingredients:**

- 1 pound lean, sliced, grilled chicken breast
- 2 cups mixed greens
- 1.5 cups sliced strawberries
- 6 tbsp light raspberry vinaigrette
- 1.5 oz crumbled goat cheese

**Directions:**

1. In a large salad bowl, mix the strawberries and cheese with the greens.

2. Toss the mixture with the vinaigrette. Divide into four salad bowls or dinner plates.

3. Divide the chicken slices among the four bowls/plates and serve.

# Tuna and Olives

**Ingredients:**

- 1/2 cup pitted olives
- 1/2 red onion, thinly sliced
- 2 tomatoes, thinly sliced
- 1/2 cucumber, thinly sliced
- 2 anchovies
- 1/3 cup olive oil
- 3 tbsp red wine vinegar
- 2 hard boiled eggs, thinly sliced
- 1 tbsp Dijon mustard
- 2 tbsp parsley
- Salt and pepper to taste
- 3 8-oz tuna fillets
- 2 tbsp canola oil
- 1 French baguette

**Directions:**

1. Mix together olives, mustard, anchovies, vinegar, and 2 tablespoons of water. Blend in a blender until smooth. Add olive oil while blending so it's emulsified.

2. Add parsley and mix with above mixture. Season with salt and pepper to taste. Set the mixture aside.

3. Brush tuna with oil and season with salt and pepper.

4. Grill tuna until cooked through—about two minutes each side.

5. Let tuna cool for five minutes, and then slice into 1/4 inch slices.

6. Cut baguette in half and brush with oil. Lightly brown on both sides—about thirty seconds.

7. Cut baguette into 4 equal pieces.

8. Put tuna and veggies on slices of bread. Top with sliced onions and egg.

9. Drizzle open faced sandwiches with the vinaigrette and serve.

## Potato Salad

**Ingredients:**

- 3 pounds of red potatoes, peeled and diced into one inch cubes
- 1/2 cup diced red onion
- 1/2 cup diced or sliced sweet pickles

- 1/2 cup diced celery
- 4 tsp Dijon mustard
- 1/4 cup sweet pickle juice
- 3/4 cup mayo
- 1/3 cup low fat buttermilk
- 1 tsp sugar
- Salt and pepper to taste
- 3 chopped boiled eggs

**Directions:**

1. Boil a large pot of water over high heat. Place potatoes in pot & cook until just tender, about 10 minutes.

2. Place boiled and drained potato pieces in a large bowl.

3. Drizzle pickle juice over potatoes and toss the mixture.

4. Let potatoes cool to room temperature.

5. Mix the rest of the ingredients in another large bowl, and fold in the potatoes with a spatula. Then refrigerate.

6. Serve after warming to room temperature.

# Italian Chicken Salad

## Ingredients:

- 2 skinless chicken breasts
- 1/2 diced red onion
- 6 sliced black olives
- 2 tbsp extra virgin olive oil
- 3 tbsp balsamic vinegar
- Sections from 1/2 orange
- 1 clove minced garlic
- Ground pepper to taste

## Directions:

1. Rub skinless chicken breasts with a crushed garlic clove.

2. Grill chicken and slice into 1/2 inch pieces. Top with sliced olives.

3. Marinate the rest of the ingredients (vinegar, olive oil, red onion, garlic, and pepper) together and drizzle the dressing on chicken.

4. Garnish with orange slices.

# Tuna in Pita Bread

**Ingredients:**

- 1 can tuna in water
- 1/2 red onion, finely chopped
- 1 cup shredded lettuce
- 1/2 cup carrots, finely chopped
- 1 jalapeno pepper, chopped
- 1 diced tomato
- 1/2 cup broccoli, finely chopped
- Fat free dressing of your choice (ranch or balsamic vinegar)
- Whole wheat pita pockets

**Directions:**

1. Mix tuna, onion, lettuce, carrots, jalapeno, tomato, and broccoli together. Toss with about a fourth cup of dressing.

2. Stuff each pita pocket with the mixture of tuna and vegetables.

# Balsamic Chicken on a Bun

**Ingredients:**

- 2 pounds cubed boneless chicken breasts
- 1/4 cup whole wheat flour
- 1/2 cup pureed broccoli
- 1/2 cup balsamic vinegar
- 1/2 tsp pepper
- 2 tsp chopped fresh basil
- 6 slices of a large tomato
- 6 tbsp brown sugar
- Dash of salt
- 3 tbs olive oil
- 1/2 cup grated mozzarella cheese
- 3 cloves garlic, minced
- 1 cup low sodium chicken broth
- 6 Ciabatta rolls

**Directions:**

1. Season chicken pieces with salt and pepper.

2. Toss chicken with flour until well coated.

3. Heat the oil in a skillet and add garlic and chicken pieces. Cook for 8-10 minutes until chicken is browned and cooked through.

4. Add the broth, vinegar, and brown sugar and vinegar.

5. Bring to a boil, then simmer 10-15 minutes on low heat.

6. Add broccoli puree and cook for another 3 minutes.

7. Open rolls and put on chicken, tomato slice, cheese pieces, and basil.

8. Bake at 350 degrees for a few minutes until the rolls crisp at the edges.

9. Put the rolls together and serve for 6.

# Super Chicken Salad

**Ingredients:**

- 6 oz. cubed chicken (breast meat is best)
- 2 leaves of lettuce
- 1/2 cup mayo
- 1 tbsp sherry vinegar
- 1 tbsp diced apple
- 1 tbsp diced celery
- 1 tbsp diced carrots
- 1 tbsp diced onion
- 1/2 tsp paprika
- 1 tbsp chopped chives
- 1/2 tsp pepper
- 1 tsp curry powder
- 15 raisins (the yellow kind)
- 2 slices of bread or one Ciabatta roll

**Directions:**

1. Combine ingredients except for lettuce in a large bowl and toss them together.

2. Open bread and lay down chicken, lettuce and the rest of the ingredients.

3. Serve warm.

# Chicken Fingers

## Ingredients:

- 1-1/4 pounds of raw chicken fingers
- 2 tbsp olive oil
- 1.5 cups Cheez-it cheddar crackers
- 1/3 cup Dijon mustard
- 1/2 tsp pepper (black)

## Directions:

1. In a blender, blend Cheez-it crackers into crumbs. Put in a bowl and stir in pepper.

2. Put tenders in mustard and then dredge them in the cracker crumbs.

3. Brush a baking pan with olive oil. Place chicken in baking pan.

4. Place oven rack in lowest part of oven and bake at 475 degrees Fahrenheit, for 15 minutes, turning once.

5. Serve warm.

# Dinner Recipes

## Tuna Steaks

**Ingredients:**

- 6 one-inch tuna steaks, about 6 oz. each
- 1/4 cup whole peppercorns
- 2 tbsp lemon juice
- 2 tbsp extra virgin olive oil
- Salt & pepper to taste
- Roasted garlic orange mayo

**Directions:**

1. Put the tuna steaks in a large bowl. Coat with oil, lemon juice, salt, and pepper.

2. Marinade the tuna for about 20 minutes.

3. Coarsely crush peppercorns and place on a big plate.

4. Dip the edges of the marinated tuna in peppercorns and then heat in a skillet over medium to high heat.

5. Cook about 5 minutes per side, adding some marinade to skillet so the steaks don't stick.

6. Top with roasted garlic orange mayo.

## Zesty Fish Tacos for Eight

**Ingredients:**

- 2 pounds of mahi-mahi
- 1.5 tsp minced garlic
- 1.5 tsp ground coriander
- 3 tbsp lime juice
- 5 tsp of chili powder
- 1/2 cup vegetable oil
- 1.5 tsp ground cumin
- Salt to taste
- 8 flour tortillas
- 1 cup Pico de Gallo—see directions below
- 1/2 cup Mexican Crema—see directions below
- Southwestern slaw—see directions below

**Directions:**

1. To make Pico de Gallo, mix together a cup of seeded, diced tomatoes, 1/2 minced Chipotle pepper, 4 tsp of minced red onion, canned, 1 tbsp sliced cilantro, 1/2 tsp red wine vinegar, and salt to taste.

2. To make the Mexican Crema, mix 2 tsp lime juice, 1/2 cup sour cream, and 1/2 tsp finely grated lime zest.

3. To make Southwestern slaw, mix together 2 tbsp minced red onion, 2 cups green cabbage, 2 tsp of chopped cilantro, 2 tsp honey, 2 tsp minced jalapeno, and 2 tsp lime juice. Add salt to taste.

4. Get a gas or charcoal grill going to temperature.

5. Cut the fish into about 16 slices.

6. Mix together oil, lime juice, chili powder, and other spices. Marinade fish with the mixture.

7. Grill the fish for about 2 minutes on each side. Fish should be cooked through.

8. Grill tortillas until they are heated through about fifteen seconds a side.

9. Place two pieces of fish in taco and top with Southwestern slaw, Pico de Gallo and Mexican Crema.

## Baked Mojo Fish

**Ingredients:**

- 1 sweet onion, large, sliced thinly
- 2 big, very ripe tomatoes, sliced thinly
- 2 tbsp minced garlic
- 3 tsp olive oil
- 1/3 cup orange juice
- 1 tsp salt
- 1/2 tsp black pepper
- 4 small fillets of fish, including tilapia or flounder

**Directions:**

1. Cook onions in a large skillet with 1 tsp olive oil for about 8 minutes, until they are soft and golden.

2. Make the Mojo sauce in a blender by mixing 2 tsp olive oil, salt, pepper, garlic, and orange juice until the mixture is smooth.

3. Cover a large baking sheet with aluminum foil and spray the aluminum foil with non-stick cooking spray.

4. Place four mounds of onions on the baking sheet. Top with half the tomatoes, the fillets and finally the rest of the tomatoes. Drizzle the Mojo sauce between each layer and on top.

5. Place on top of the oven and bake at 400 degrees Fahrenheit for 8-10 minutes. Serve hot.

## DASH Pasta Primavera

**Ingredients:**
- 1 box bow tie pasta (12 oz.)
- 1 cup chicken broth
- 1 bag frozen Italian veggies
- 1/2 cup Parmesan cheese, grated
- 3 tbsp fresh basil, chopped
- 2 tsp minced garlic

**Directions:**

1. Cook pasta per package directions until the pasta is al dente.

2. In a skillet, sauté garlic in olive oil for about 30 seconds.

3. Add broth and vegetables to skillet and cook until tender, about 8 minutes.

4. Stir in pasta, 2 tbsp basil and half the Parmesan cheese.

5. Top with rest of basil and parmesan cheese.

6. Serve in a large serving bowl (serves 4).

## Delicious Pasta with Pumpkin

**Ingredients:**

- 1/2 cup diced butternut squash
- 1 tbsp minced garlic
- 4 tsp chopped macadamia nuts
- 3/4 cup pumpkin, canned
- 2 tbsp concentrated pomegranate
- 1 tbsp chopped shallots

- 2 tbsp extra virgin olive oil
- 1 cup vegetable stock
- Pinch of sea salt
- Pinch of cinnamon
- Pinch of ground pepper

**Directions:**

1. In a large skillet, sauté garlic and onions and garlic in olive oil until onions are translucent.

2. Sauté butternut squash until tender.

3. Add vegetable stock, cinnamon, canned pumpkin, salt, and pepper. Cook thoroughly.

4. Cook pasta until al dente and add to pumpkin sauce.

5. Divide mixture into four separate bowls.

6. Top each bowl with a teaspoon each of macadamia nuts and a half tablespoon of pomegranate.

# Ham and Spaghetti Alfredo

**Ingredients:**

- 1 box of spaghetti (8 oz.)
- 1/2 pound cubed ham pieces
- 1/4 cup Parmesan cheese, grated
- 10 oz. of light Alfredo sauce
- 2 cups chunked broccoli
- 1/4 tsp red pepper flakes

**Directions:**

1. In a large pot, cook spaghetti until it is al dente.

2. Add broccoli and cook for a little bit more then drain. Keep the mixture warm.

3. In a saucepan, add Alfredo sauce, ham, and pepper flakes and heat until it is warm. Toss the two mixtures together.

4. Place the pasta dish in four different serving plates.

5. Sprinkle each with Parmesan cheese and pepper.

# Sausage and Linguine

## Ingredients:

- 1 pound of hot Italian sausage, pork or turkey
- 1 pound of sweet Italian sausage, pork or turkey
- 1 green pepper, diced
- 1 large onion, diced
- 1 tbsp minced garlic
- 2 red peppers, diced
- 1/4 cup extra virgin olive oil
- 6 ripe plum tomatoes, each cut into eight pieces
- 1 cup prepared marinara sauce
- 1/2 cup red wine, dry
- 1 pound cooked linguine

## Directions:

1. Cut sausages into 1/2 inch slices.

2. In a large skillet, brown sausages in olive oil. Transfer sausages to a large heavy pot.

3. Add onion and garlic. Simmer over low heat and then add peppers and increase the heat to medium.

4. Stir in tomatoes, marinara sauce, parsley, red wine, and salt &pepper to taste.

5. Simmer mixture for about thirty minutes.

6. Pour over the linguine and garnish with 2 tbsp parsley.

## Baked Rigatoni

**Ingredients:**

- 2 sweet Italian sausages with casings removed
- 2 hot Italian sausages with casings removed
- 2 tbsp olive oil
- 12 oz sliced mozzarella (make 6 slices and dice the rest)
- 2 diced tomatoes
- One box of rigatoni pasta (12 oz.)
- 2 cup prepared marinara sauce
- 1 tsp dried oregano
- 1/2 cup coarsely torn basil leaves
- 1/4 tsp hot red pepper flakes
- Salt to taste
- Pepper to taste

**Directions:**

1. In a heavy pot, heat oil and add sausages. Cook for about 12 minutes, breaking them up as you cook.

2. Transfer sausages into a large bowl using a slotted spoon.

3. Cook pasta in boiling pot of water until al dente, about 12 minutes.

4. Mix sausages with the marinara sauce and the rest of the ingredients except sliced mozzarella.

5. Put a light amount of oil in a large baking pan. Toss pasta and sausage sauce and put in baking pan. Top with the slices of mozzarella.

6. Bake until pasta is completely heated through, about 20 minutes.

## Farfalle Pasta with Peas

**Ingredients:**

- 1 pound Farfalle pasta
- 1.5 cups cherry tomatoes, each cut in half
- 1/4 cup lemon vinaigrette dressing
- 1/4 cup fresh parsley
- 3/4 cup frozen peas
- Salt & pepper to taste

**Directions:**

1. Cook pasta, drain and cool.

2. Mix with the rest of the ingredients and add salt and pepper to taste.

## Spaghetti and Tuna

**Ingredients:**

- 1 can tuna in water (5 oz.), drained
- 1/2 pound spaghetti, cooked
- 6 green olives, chopped
- 1-1/4 cups spaghetti sauce, prepared
- 1 tbsp extra virgin olive oil
- 1 onion, chopped

- 2 tbsp capers
- Salt & red pepper to taste

## Directions:

1. Cook pasta and drain. Put back over the stove on low heat.

2. In another pot, cook onion in oil for about a minute. Then add olives, spaghetti sauce, and capers. Bring to a boil and then simmer it.

3. Cut tuna into small flakes. Add to the sauce. Cook for another minute.

4. Toss the spaghetti with the sauce and add salt & pepper to taste.

## Ham and Pea Linguine

## Ingredients:

- 5 oz thickly sliced ham without visible fat, cubed into 1/2 inch cubes
- 1 pound linguine pasta; (mix spinach linguine with plain linguine)
- 1 cup thawed or cooked peas
- 1 medium onion, chopped

- 3 tbsp olive oil
- 2 garlic cloves, minced
- 2 tbsp butter
- Salt & pepper to taste

**Directions:**

1. Cook pasta in boiling water until the pasta is al dente. Drain and keep back a cup of cooking water.

2. Using a saucepan, heat onion and garlic over medium heat with oil, about 3 minutes.

3. Melt butter in the pan and add ham and peas. Cook until the mixture is heated through, about 3 minutes.

4. Add sauce to pasta and season with salt & pepper to taste.

5. Add some extra cooking water so that a light sauce is created. Serve immediately.

# Chapter 6: Seven-Day DASH Diet Menu

This is a sample of what a week on the DASH diet would look like. The recipes are easy to make and are healthy for the entire family. You can make substitutions if you like, keeping an eye out for the potassium and sodium concentrations of what you're eating.

Learn to like less salt and encourage your children to eat foods that are lower in salt because salt is an acquired taste that you can get out of after a period of time.

### Day One

**Breakfast:** Cheesy Eggs, one slice whole wheat pita, 1/2 grapefruit.

1. Cheesy eggs are made with a whole egg, two egg whites and fat free milk—all sautéed in a nonstick pan.

2. Mix in an ounce of low fat cheese, 2 sundried tomatoes (chopped) and 1 chopped green onion.

3. Scramble this and put inside the pita bread.

**Lunch:** Stuffed red pepper with couscous and chickpeas, one cup fat free milk.

1. Make the stuffed red pepper by cooking 1/4 cup couscous in 1/3 cup chicken broth.

2. Continue by hollowing out the pepper.

3. Dice the top of the pepper and add it to cooked couscous.

4. Add a fourth cup drained, canned chickpeas, 1/4 cup diced, dried apricots, 1/4 tsp cumin and 4 drops Tabasco sauce.

5. Mix all ingredients including 3/4 cup minced parsley and a squirt of lemon.

6. Stuff the pepper and broil pepper for a few minutes until charred.

**Dinner:** Stir fry with fresh mango and 1/2 cup low fat frozen yogurt.

1. Marinate a cup of extra firm diced tofu in a tablespoon of low salt soy sauce, 2 tsp lime juice and 3 drops of Tabasco sauce, a teaspoon of sugar and 1/2 tsp sesame oil for about 10-60 minutes.

2. Heat a wok and add a cup of sugar snap peas, tofu and marinade.

3. Add 1/3 cup of chicken broth and cook until liquid is nearly gone.

4. Add 1.5 cups instant whole grain rice, 1/2 cup diced mango, and 1/4 cup of green onions, minced.

5. Cook in wok until flavors are blended.

6. Snacks: one apple; 6 whole grain crackers.

## Day Two

**Breakfast:** Muesli, Breakfast Shake.

1.  Mix 3/4 cup muesli with 3/4 cup fat free milk.

2.  Add half of a diced medium apple and two tbsp of dried currants or raisins.

3.  Make the shake with a blender by blending a half of one banana, a whole orange (peeled), 1/4 cup fat free milk, 1/2 tbsp honey, a couple of ice cubes and a pinch of nutmeg.

4.  Drink cold.

**Lunch:** Shrimp quesadillas, sweet Jicama salad and one pear.

1.  Make quesadillas by mixing a half oz of low fat smoked mozzarella cheese, grated, with 3 oz diced, cooked shrimp.

2.  Add 1/2 tsp cumin, 1/4 cup chopped red onion, one chopped plum tomato without seeds, and one diced jalapeno.

3. Spread mixture on two whole wheat tortillas and heat in a nonstick skillet open faced.

4. Fold, cut in wedges and serve.

5. Make the Jicama salad by peeling and slicing a quarter pound of Jicama so that it is in 1/4 inch pieces. Put in large bowl.

6. Put in half of a fennel bulb sliced into half moons.

7. Slice a fourth of an onion into small slices and add to mixture.

8. Squeeze the juice of a small seedless tangerine over mixture and sprinkle a pinch of salt and pepper to taste.

**Dinner:** Salmon with ginger, artichoke heart salad and a whole wheat roll with jelly. Sliced strawberries for dessert. Drink a cup of fat free milk.

1. Make salmon with ginger by marinating 4 oz of salmon for 15 minutes in a marinade of 1/4 cup soy sauce, 2 tbsp balsamic vine-

gar, 1/2 tsp sesame oil and a 2 inch piece of peeled ginger root, grated.

2. Heat up a nonstick skillet with a tsp of olive oil. Sauté the salmon until cooked, about a minute per side.

3. Sprinkle salmon with sesame seeds.

4. Garnish with minced green onion.

5. To make the artichoke heart salad, toss together 1/4 head of romaine lettuce (chopped), 1/4 cucumber (sliced), 2 tomatoes (diced), and 4 ounces of artichoke hearts.

6. Make a dressing with a minced garlic clove, 2 tsp olive oil and the juice of one lemon.

7. Add 1/2 tsp dried oregano, a pinch of salt and a pinch of pepper.

8. Snacks: 3/4 cup unsalted pretzels and 1/3 c raisins.

## Day Three

**Breakfast:** Hash Browned Potatoes with peppers and onions and scrambled eggs; whole grain toast; 1 orange; decaf latte with fat free milk.

1. To make hash browns with peppers and onions, sauté two small red-skinned potatoes, 1/4 medium onion, 1/4 diced green pepper in a tsp of olive oil.

2. Add a pinch of pepper and stir until browned.

3. Add 1/4 cup chicken broth and keep covered for three minutes.

4. In another bowl, take one egg, one egg white and 1 tbsp fat free milk, whisked together.

5. Pour eggs into vegetables and cook the combination until firm—about 20 minutes.

6. Season to taste with salt and pepper.

**Lunch:** Corn soup with Poblano black beans, baked tortilla chips, cucumber and orange salad, 1 cup fat free milk.

1. To make the soup, sauté in 1/2 tsp olive oil, 1/4 of a white onion (diced), 1/2 of a Poblano pepper, diced, 2 cloves minced garlic and 1/4 tsp cumin, 1/4 tsp dried oregano for 2 minutes.

2. Add a half can of rinsed black beans, 1/2 cup corn, 1 tsp balsamic vinegar and a cup of chicken stock.

3. Cook for about 8 minutes and add a tbsp of parmesan cheese.

4. To make the salad, slice 1/2 large cucumber with an orange.

5. Squeeze on a squirt of lime, 1/4 tsp chili powder and a tsp of toasted pumpkin seeds.

**Dinner:** Chicken with raisins and olives, one cup melon balls.

1. To make chicken, sauté a quarter cup of uncooked long grain rice with a tsp of olive oil. The rice should pop after 2 minutes.

2. Add a half cup of salsa, 1/2 cup of chicken stock, 1 piece of chicken breast, halved, 3/4 cup baby carrots, 2 tbsp pitted, chopped green olives and 2 tbsp raisins.

3. Add 1/2 tsp ground cinnamon. Simmer in pan and cover tightly.

4. Bake in a 375 degree oven until the moisture is absorbed, about 20-25 minutes.

5. Top with a couple of tablespoons of cilantro, chopped.

6. Toss everything together before serving.

7. Snacks: 1 cup fat free yogurt; 1.5 cups plain popcorn.

# Day Four

**Breakfast:** Maple Prune Oatmeal; Iced latte; 1 cup fat free milk.

1.  To make oatmeal, take 3/4 cup of rolled oats and mix with 3/4 cup fat free milk.

2.  Cook until bubbling for up to 8 minutes, stirring the whole time.

3.  Stir in a quarter cup of apple cider and 2 diced fresh plums.

4.  Add 1/4 cup diced prunes and a table-spoon of maple syrup.

5.  Sprinkle the whole thing with cinnamon.

**Lunch:** Lentils with vegetables; a cup of grapes.

1.  To make lentil mixture, take 3/4 cup green lentils and mix with 2 large bay leaves, 4 cups water and 1 tsp dried oregano.

2.  Simmer 20 minutes until lentils are tender.

3.  Drain off liquid and combine lentils with diced insides of two scooped out tomatoes,

1 oz crumbled feta, 1 cup arugula, chopped, 2 tsp thyme, and 2 tsp vinegar.

4. Stuff this mixture with tomato outsides and garnish with thyme.

**Dinner:** Spaghetti with Tuna, Escarole and Potatoes, 1/2 low fat frozen yogurt.

1. To make spaghetti, sauté half an onion, diced, along with 1 clove minced garlic, 1/2 tsp anchovy paste and 1/2 of a chipotle chili, minced, for a couple of minutes.

2. Add a cup of freshly chopped plum tomatoes, 1 tsp drained capers. Sauté another 2 minutes.

3. Put in a cup of chopped fresh spinach and 3 ounces of fresh tuna cut in cubes.

4. Cook for 90 seconds. Sprinkle with 1/2 tbsp dried marjoram.

5. Serve over 2 oz whole wheat spaghetti, cooked.

6. For Escarole and Potatoes, add 2 large cloves slivered garlic, sautéed in a teaspoon of olive oil for ten seconds.

7.  Add two cups escarole (cut into one inch pieces) and a quarter pound of red skinned new potatoes, diced. Sauté two minutes.

8.  Add 1/4 tsp pepper, 1/4 cup slivered mint and 1/2 cup chicken stock.

9.  Cook on low for five minutes.

10. Snacks: 1/4 cup dried fruit mixture; 6 whole grain crackers.

## Day Five

**Breakfast:** Yogurt with fresh strawberries; granola with toasted almonds; 1/2 medium grapefruit.

1.  To make yogurt with strawberries, mix a cup of quartered fresh strawberries with a tsp of brown sugar.

2.  Add this mixture to a bowl of fat free yogurt, strawberry or plain.

3.  For granola, mix a quarter cup of slivered toasted almonds with 1/4 cup low fat granola.

**Lunch:** Polenta cake with rosemary; mine-strone soup.

1. To make polenta cake, sauté 3 large cloves garlic (minced) in a tsp of olive oil.

2. Add 1/2 cup water, 1/2 cup fat free milk, 1/2 tsp salt and black pepper.

3. Add a fourth of a tsp of dried rosemary. Boil and reduce heat.

4. Add 1/2 cup quick cooking polenta. Stir 5-8 minutes.

5. When polenta is thick add a cup of corn and mix with polenta.

6. Stir in 1.5 oz grated Romano cheese along with 1/4 cup chopped chives.

7. Pour into pie tin to sit for 10 minutes.

8. Garnish with a half tsp fresh minced rosemary.

**Dinner:** Thai subs; spinach and mushroom salad; vinaigrette dressing; 1 c fresh fruit salad.

1. To make Thai subs, mix 8 cloves of minced garlic, 6 halves of Serrano peppers, 2 cups vegetable stock, 1/4 cup fish sauce, the juice of one half of a lime, and one tsp sugar.

2. Slice thinly 1/2 small eggplant lengthwise, 1/2 eggplant, 1/2 zucchini and 1/2 summer squash.

3. Marinate the vegetables along with two large tops of Portobello mushrooms for 15-60 minutes.

4. Grill the vegetables until slightly charred.

5. Slice mushroom caps and layer vegetables on 2 whole wheat hot dog buns.

6. Snacks: 1 cup low fat chocolate milk; 1 banana.

## Day Six

**Breakfast:** Oatmeal and steamed apples; tangerine.

1. To make oatmeal, take 1/2 cup rolled oats and cook according to package directions.

2. Core and peel one apple and dice.

3. Microwave apples until warm and soft, about 1 minute.

4. Add 1/2 tsp sugar to apples and add mixture to oatmeal in a bowl.

5. Sprinkle a dash of cinnamon on top and eat.

**Lunch:** Tomato Soup; Grilled Cheese Sandwich.

1. To make tomato soup, put together these ingredients: 2 tsp butter, 2 tbsp olive oil, 2 cups diced onions, 1 tbsp garlic, minced, 1/2 tsp ground allspice, 1/3 cup fresh dill, 6 cup chicken broth, 1 tsp sugar, 2 large cans peeled, chopped, drained tomatoes, salt and pepper to taste, sour cream for garnish.

2. Melt butter and oil over low heat in big pot.

3. Add onions and cook for 10 minutes.

4. Add garlic and continue cooking.

5. Sprinkle the allspice into the mixture.

6. Add half of the dill and continue cooking over low heat for about five minutes.

7. Add broth, tomatoes, sugar and spices, cooking for twenty minutes.

8. Puree the whole thing in a food processor and then transfer back to the pot, adding the rest of the dill.

9. Serve with sour cream over each bowl.

**Dinner:** Asian salmon; 1 cup milk; mixed summer vegetables.

1. To make Asian salmon, marinate salmon fillets in a mixture of 2 cloves garlic (minced), 2 tbsp soy sauce, 1/4 cup pineapple juice, 1 inch peeled chopped ginger. Marinate for about 60 minutes.

2. Put each salmon fillet in tin foil and sprinkle each with some pepper and sesame oil before sealing.

3. Bake for around ten minutes on a side in the oven.

4. For the mixed summer vegetables, mix a cup of sliced okra, a cup of sliced zucchini, and a sliced green and red pepper.

5. Steam the entire group of vegetables in a steamer and serve with a fourth of a tsp of salt and pepper to taste.

6. Snacks: One plum; 1/2 cup low fat yogurt.

## Day Seven

**Breakfast:** Peach Fromage; whole wheat toast with marmalade.

1. For the Peach Fromage, use 8 peaches or nectarines, 1/2 cup honey, 1/2 tsp cinnamon, 1/4 tsp ground ginger, 8 oz mascarpone cheese.

2. Heat the honey in a small sauce pan. Add cinnamon and ginger. Put aside.

3. Cut fruit into halves and quarters and put into a serving dish.

4. Put fromage on the fruit by the teaspoonful until well covered.

5.  Drizzle the mixture with warm honey mixture and serve right away.

**Lunch:** Indian Carrot Soup; Sliced Apple; whole grain toast with spray of liquid butter.

1.  To make the Indian Carrot Soup, heat a tsp of mustard seeds until they splutter and then add one chopped onion in a small amount of olive oil.

2.  Add 3 cups chopped carrots, 1/2 tsp curry powder, 1 inch chopped ginger root, peeled, 1/2 tsp chili powder and black pepper to taste.

3.  Add 4 cups vegetable stock and cook until carrots are cooked.

4.  Blend all ingredients into a blender and then garnish with a dollop of lean sour cream, lime juice squirt and chopped coriander.

**Dinner:** 3 ounces of grilled chicken breast with lemon squirt on it; pasta and veggie salad.

1. To make the pasta and veggie salad, heat up 1/2 cup chicken broth with a clove of minced garlic, 2 onions, chopped, and one can of chopped tomatoes.

2. Cook five minutes and then add some mushrooms, zucchini and one hot pepper, all chopped.

3. Cook for an additional five minutes. Then add 1 tsp fresh basil and 1 tsp oregano and then add freshly cooked pasta.

4. Chill in refrigerator for an hour before serving.

So for seven days, you've eaten the DASH diet and you have plenty of recipes to start your DASH diet with. Keep them on file in your computer or on recipe cards so you can mix and match your meals. By all means, eat what you like because that's how you go about losing weight and lowering your blood pressure.

# Conclusion

High blood pressure is so common that almost a third of Americans suffer from it and scores more have prehypertension, which means their blood pressure is above desirable but not so high they need medication. If this is you, the DASH diet is a perfect way to lower your blood pressure and eat healthier for a longer life.

While the DASH diet is technically a way to lower blood pressure, it is actually a way of living that you and your family can stick with for the rest of your lives. Rather than being a "diet" that you go on and then go off when you've reached your target goals, the DASH diet really is something you incorporate into everyday living.

Although the DASH diet strictly is all about blood pressure reduction, this guide talked about several different things you can do to lower blood pressure. These things included:

- Maintaining a healthy weight with a BMI of 25 or less, but not lower than 18.

- Exercising 30 minutes a day.

- Keeping sodium content to less than 1500 mg sodium per day.

- Increasing potassium in your diet through foods that contain potassium.

These are all good ways to lower blood pressure but doing them all in the context of a DASH diet make them really powerful when it comes to overall health and lowered blood pressure. A certain percentage of those on medication for hypertension will be able to get off some of them or all of them. Practically all those with prehypertension will have normal blood pressure or at least won't elevate to high blood pressure and require medications.

People who eat the DASH diet and follow the above recommendations have a much greater chance of having a long life free of heart disease, stroke, vision loss, peripheral vascular disease and kidney damage. These are the complications of high blood pressure that would be at a lesser incidence when eating the DASH diet.

The DASH diet does not specifically address cholesterol but this issue needs to be looked at as well, especially if you have a family history of high cholesterol. The DASH diet is low in dietary cholesterol so it should help keep high cholesterol at bay but you should have your cholesterol checked after you've been on the DASH diet for a few months.

If your cholesterol is high, you may need to be on cholesterol lowering drugs. The guidelines for cholesterol are having total cholesterol of less than 200 mg/dL and an LDL or "bad" cholesterol of less than 100 mg/dL. Ideally the "good" cholesterol should be greater than 50 mg/dL and the triglycerides should be less than 150 mg/dL. All of these lipids interact to create either a favorable or unfavorable cholesterol profile. While some of it can be addressed in what you eat, 70 percent of cholesterol products are produced by the body so medications may need to be addressed.

The DASH diet may be the perfect choice for those who suffer from metabolic syndrome, a poorly understood medical condition that leads to heart disease and stroke. It consists of these components:

- High blood pressure

- Insulin resistance and possibly type II diabetes

- Truncal obesity (obesity around the middle of the waist)

- Sedentary Lifestyle

- Excessive ability to clot blood

If these kinds of people followed the DASH diet and exercised so that they lost weight, the insulin resistance would diminish and the individual would potentially be spared the complications of the disease, including the serious ones.

The guide included a number of recipes as a guide to how you might eat on the DASH diet. To make this really part of your lifestyle, see if you can adapt some of your own recipes by substituting fat free dairy products with whole fat products, by reducing salt and adding spices, and by using lean poultry or fish instead of beef when you cook. Add fruits or veggie snacks instead of potato chips and white flour products when snacking so you can feel full most of the time without resorting to foods that only harm you.

The DASH diet was what inspired today's food pyramid. What it means is that, by eating the DASH diet, you are eating what experts recommend as the ideal diet, even if you didn't have high blood pressure. Because the DASH diet doesn't really keep track of calories—only servings—all you need to know is how much of any one thing constitutes a serving and really stick to one serving if you mean to eat one serving.

Remember that it doesn't take much meat to constitute a serving so you can eat more than one serving of meat per meal to add up to the 6 servings or less per day of lean meat per day. If you stick to the foods recommended on the diet and know your serving sizes, the caloric content will average out the right number of calories on any given day. At first, you might have to consciously count out the servings to make sure you're getting enough and not too much but, over time, the DASH diet will become second nature and you'll have meal plans all laid out without difficulty.

Try the DASH diet for better health and a longer life. It is sure to be the way people eat whenever they suffer from high blood pressure or obesity. It is what many government agencies looking to recommend better health for everyone are recommending. Try it for six months with before and after blood pressure readings, and before and after weight checks to see if, in fact, it is something you can live with for a long time to come.

www.ingramcontent.com/pod-product-compliance
Lightning Source LLC
Chambersburg PA
CBHW071158280526
45787CB00002B/539